IT'S YOUR LIFE – EXERCISE FOR ALL AGES

Professor Norman Ratcliffe

A catalogue record for this book is available from the British Library

ISBN: 978-1-907962-63-9

Published by Cranmore Publications

www.cranmorepublications.co.uk

This book is dedicated to my parents whose undying faith in my academic capabilities allowed me to pursue a scientific career. My gratitude also goes to my sister, Teri King, whose success as an author and constant encouragement and advice were such sources of inspiration. Thanks too to my many friends for tolerating so many mealtime discussions on health and diet as well as the unsolicited advice given to them!

Finally, I wish to thank Dr. Duncan McLaren of Swansea Metropolitan University for his outstanding enthusiasm and imagination during creation of sections of this book as well as Doreen Montgomery of Rupert Crew Ltd for her patient and helpful comments of the manuscript.

"IT'S YOUR LIFE"

THE AUTHOR

- **Professor Norman Ratcliffe** is a founder member of a team that recently discovered a new antibiotic potentially capable of curing MRSA and *Clostridium difficile*. This work was presented to Prince Phillip at St. James's Palace, London and was the subject of major media attention in the UK on ITV News and in many leading newspapers, including the Wall Street Journal, around the World. He is a Fellow of the Royal Society of Medicine and has previously run a "Health Alert" blood-testing company. He has published over 200 books and research papers on immunology, cancer invasion, influenza, tropical diseases and MRSA. He played squash for Wales, ran the London Marathon at the age of 50 and works-out regularly in the gym.

- **Professor Ratcliffe** retired recently after 25 years as a University Research Professor. He decided to finally complete "It's Your Life" after 5 years work in order to help the many people who are confused about health and fitness issues and who have constantly been asking his advice.

"IT'S YOUR LIFE"

THE SERIES

Professor Norman Ratcliffe's comprehensive book on health is: *It's Your Life: End the confusion from inconsistent health advice:*

www.cranmorepublications.co.uk/6

This book will often be referred to as IYL. Alongside this comprehensive book there is a series of smaller *It's Your Life: End the confusion from inconsistent health advice* books; this book is the fifth in the series. The aim of the series is to give advice to people in specific areas; all of the areas covered in the series are also included in IYL. The series is as follows:

It's Your Life – A Healthy Diet Made Easy

www.cranmorepublications.co.uk/61

It's Your Life – Avoiding Harmful Chemicals in Your Food

www.cranmorepublications.co.uk/62

It's Your Life – Avoid the Cocktail Effect of Harmful Chemicals in Your Body

www.cranmorepublications.co.uk/63

It's Your Life – Vitamins and Supplements For All Ages

www.cranmorepublications.co.uk/64

It's Your Life – Exercise For All Ages

www.cranmorepublications.co.uk/65

The main advice arising from IYL has also been summarised in:

117 Health Tips: A quick guide for a healthy life

www.cranmorepublications.co.uk/7

Contents

CHAPTER 1

EXERCISE

Basic Introduction

DO I REALLY HAVE TO EXERCISE?

WHY BOTHER? Every health article urges us to take regular exercise to become fit thus avoiding **heart problems** and strengthening the bones to prevent age-related diseases such as **osteoporosis** (weakened bones that easily fracture, especially in post-menopausal women). Other benefits from regular exercise are the maintenance of **muscle tone**, the control of **body weight** to lessen the stress on joints, and a reduction in the likelihood of **diabetes** developing. If you suffer from stiffness, weakness and lack of energy, this is not an inevitable consequence of old age (say 50+) but probably due to **inactivity**.

*Advantages of Regular Exercise
Controls body weight
Reduces risk of high blood pressure
Reduces risk of heart problems
Reduces risk of strokes

Reduces risk of diabetes
Strengthens bones
Strengthens resistance to disease
Tones muscles
Increases energy levels
Retains joint flexibility
Increases sexual activity
Delays aging and frailty
Protects against Alzheimer's?
Improves mental outlook
Reduces stress

*See, for example, references 134 and 135

Figure 1, below, shows ABSOLUTELY CLEARLY how a simple exercise such as walking daily can reduce premature death (Graph modified from Hakim and colleagues (see reference 136)

- The graph shows that when retired men walked less than 1 mile per day (< 1 mile) then after 12 years over 40.5% of them had died from all causes. This 40.5% death rate was nearly twice that at 23.8% of another group of retired men who walked more than 2 miles per day (> 2 mile).

- Of these dead men, 13.4% and 5.3% died of cancer, respectively, in the < 1 mile versus the > 2mile groups, while 6.6% and 2.1% died of heart disease/strokes in these same groups.

- In other words, death, cancer and heart disease/stroke rates were 2 to 3 times higher in men who walked less than 1 mile per day compared with those who walked more than 2 miles per day.

Figure 1. Showing how walking regularly can reduce death rates of retired men

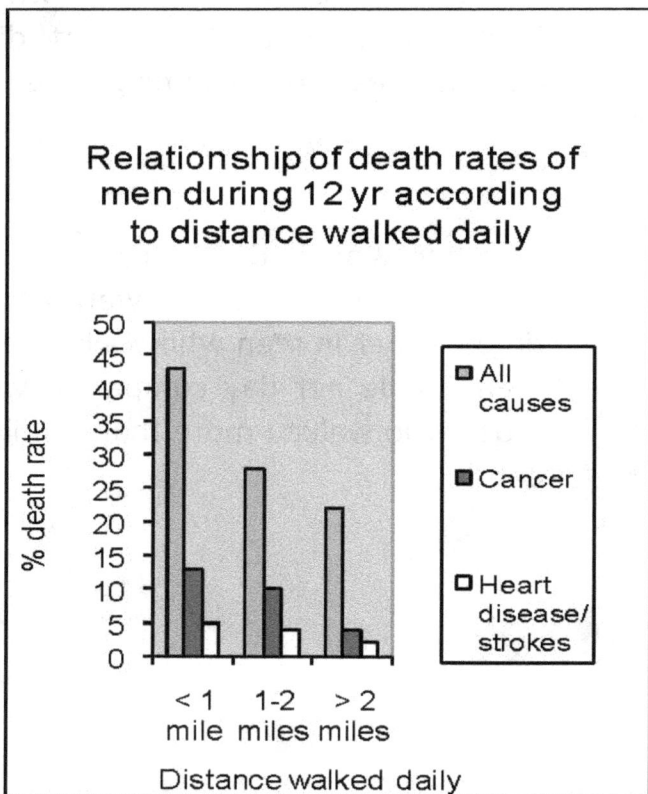

Relationship of death rates of men during 12 yr according to distance walked daily

You will be amazed how much better you feel once you begin a regular exercise regimen. Regular exercise will help to maintain your mental health and avoid physical problems developing as well as relieving the stress and strain of everyday life.

IT IS ESSENTIAL IF YOU HAVE NOT TAKEN REGULAR EXERCISE FOR A LONG TIME, AND ESPECIALLY IF YOU ARE GROSSLY OVERWEIGHT, THAT YOU CONSULT YOUR DOCTOR BEFORE EMBARKING ON ANY NEW STRENUOUS EXERCISE REGIMEN

CHAPTER 2

EXERCISE

For Gym Lovers

TO GYM OR NOT TO GYM
THAT IS THE QUESTION?

Exercise

- I believe **that you either are or are not a gym person**. Despite this, the most popular advice suggested by many health gurus is **"get ye to a gym"** and start heaving weights around or doing aerobics. I have many friends who simply could **never** be induced to go into a gym and look at me aghast that at my time of life (or any other) I should bother to go to such a place.

- **OK, the gym is not for you.** So miss out this section and go to "Alternative Types of Exercise" (see Chapter 3).

- **For gym people.** Sometimes individuals go to the gym, take one look and never return because they feel **intimidated or self-conscious** in some way. I have visited gyms around the world and can confirm that they are **rarely filled** with perfect physical specimens! Quite the opposite in many cases. So give it a try. **Your first experience** in the gym will very much depend upon the instructor showing you around, as well as the type of gym that you are visiting. Many instructors tend to be young and often very fit and, unfortunately, unaware of the intimidation that can be felt by the novice. They also spend too much time on their stations and not enough keeping an eye on novices using the gym who may be too shy to ask for help.

Figure 1. Avoid gyms full of enormous steroid freaks as you will be intimidated and probably receive scant attention from the instructors

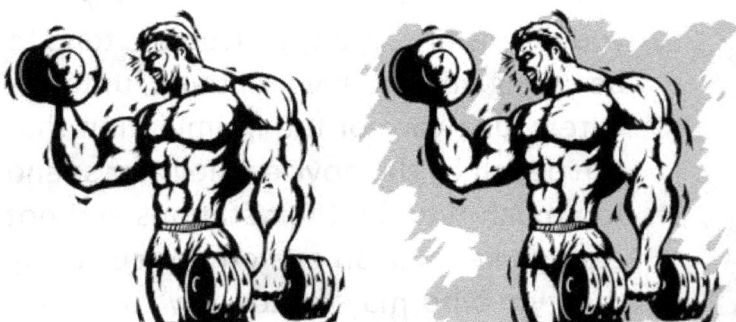

- The **worst type of gym** for a first-timer is where everyone is in their 20-40s, wearing all the latest high–tech gear, and containing a high percentage of posers and/or enormous steroid freaks lifting enormous weights and grunting.

- Try going to **a YMCA or Local Authority Gym** because these tend to contain more of a mix of ages with posers going to the more expensive establishments with larger mirrors all around.

- Try and find someone to train with you as **"Gym Buddies"** are worth their weight in gold and often can correct your technique and provide much-needed motivation. Your gym buddy could be a friend who also wishes to begin training. Believe me, there is nothing like a gym buddy to persuade you to go to the gym on a cold, dark and wet night after a hard days work!

Figure 2. Try and find somebody (your gym buddy) to train with as they will provide motivation and improve your progress

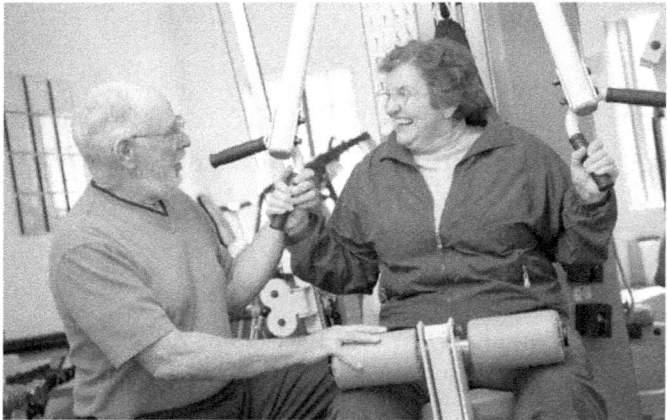

- Ok, you are in the gym at last, so what do you do? One of the instructors should show you how to use all the aerobics equipment (rowing machines, bicycles, treadmills, steppers etc) as well as all the other confusing machines and the free weights (dumbbells and barbells). This is your so-called "**induction**" but don't worry, you will not have to remember everything. Subsequently, he/she **should provide you** with a detailed **written workout programme** designed uniquely for your requirements. A gym should only allow you to train if you have had an induction in the use of the equipment.

Figure 3. An instructor should show you how to use the equipment (induction) and provide you with a training programme

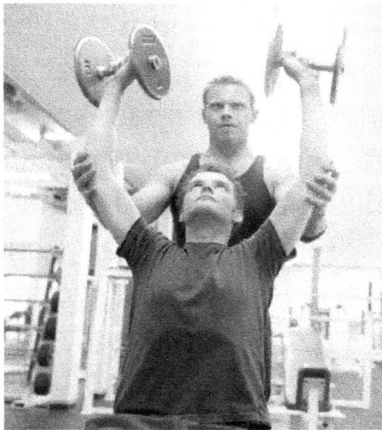

- **Design of your work-out programme.** Ideally, this should contain a mix of aerobic exercise to strengthen the heart, lungs and circulation as well as some weights to strengthen the muscles of the body. The usual advice is to slowly work up to **three 30 minutes aerobic sessions per week** as well as about the same amount of time for weight training. However, these are **just guidelines and should be modified at regular intervals by an instructor**. Personally, I believe that the cycle, rower and the cross trainer (a devilish machine designed to work both the upper body as well as the legs) are better than the treadmill as less impact and wear occurs on the joints. Aerobic machines can be incredibly **boring** and some gyms run **Cycle Spinning Classes** which involve a semi-circle of static cycles around an instructor on a cycle in the centre who simulates hill climbs and flat racing with you. **Buying a padded seat for these static**

cycles is advisable. These spinning classes are good fun and you are usually inspired by an excellent choice of music.

Figure 4. A typical spin class with static cycles

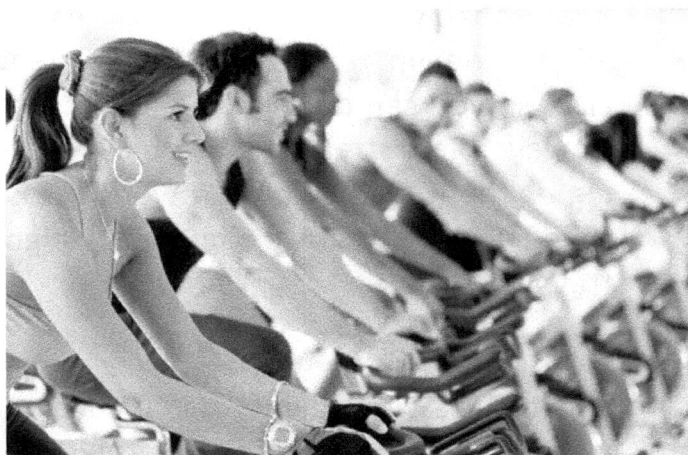

- During the spinning class, you set your own pace (but are actively encouraged by the instructor) and time and calories are rapidly used up. You can burn 800 or more calories in a 50 min session and actually enjoy yourself. A friend of mine once attended a gym in which the cycles had individual screens (like the seats in modern jet planes) on which porno films could be accessed. I guess that he burnt some extra calories in this particular workout! You probably will not have much energy left for weight training after a spinning class so you can do this on another day. However, less strenuous aerobic exercising on the treadmill, bike, rower or cross trainer can be followed by your weight training.

- For starting with weights, if you have not already warmed up with an aerobic session then begin with some gentle aerobic exercise, such as walking or cycling for 5-10 min. Having warmed up, gently, **stretch** the limbs and back, without jerking, as shown in wall charts around the gym and by an instructor. You are now ready to strengthen your body with weights.

Figure 5. Emphasising the necessity of stretching the body prior to strenuous exercise

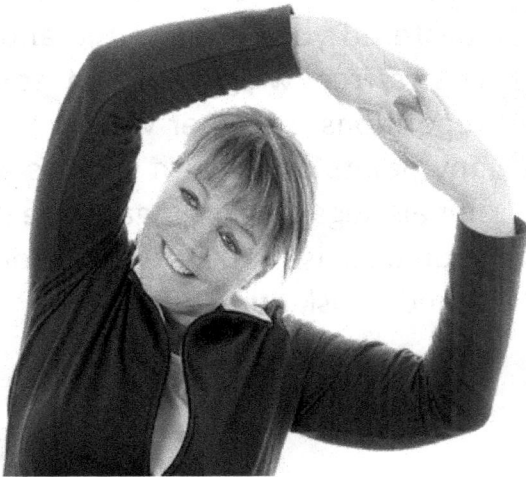

- **Exercising with weights.** First, you have to decide exactly **what you wish to achieve** with the weights. Do you want to generally strengthen the whole body or are there particular parts of your body that you wish to improve?

- **Probably the best strategy** is to train all the main muscle groups in the body each week and then after a few weeks, having mastered your programme and the machines/free weights, fit in some extra repetitions or higher weight to focus on any points of concern such as the abdominals, legs or arms. Again, the instructor should advise you here so do not be frightened to **ask questions**.

- **One possible programme** would be to train Mondays, Wednesdays and Fridays beginning with a 20-30 min aerobic exercise (row, cycle, jog etc) and then followed by a 20-30 min weights session. Finish off by stretching and/or cycling or rowing etc for 5-10 min.

•	**Mondays, aerobics then train back and biceps**
•	**Wednesdays, aerobics then train chest and abdominal muscles**
•	**Fridays, aerobics then train legs, shoulders and triceps**
•	**Weekends, walk/cycle or sport [a]**

[a] **Try to do some form of exercise at the weekend, even if it is just to stay away from the pub or television for a while. Taking part in some active sport is ideal and can count as an aerobic session. One of the best exercises for ALL AGES is to cycle instead of using the car as this not only burns calories but also saves money and the environment.**

- For weights, generally speaking, start with one or two sets of 6+ repetitions and work up to three sets of 10 repetitions with each exercise before increasing the weight.

- For **toning**, the weights should be relatively **light** with higher numbers of repetitions of 15-20. For gaining **muscle bulk,** heavier weights with fewer repetitions of 6-8 should be used. Again, decide which body part you want to improve and ask the instructor to help you.

Things to remember

1. **Always warm up and warm down** for 5-10 min before and after exercise.

2. **Sip water regularly** during your work-out to avoid dehydration and subsequent weakness. Aim to drink about one small

bottle of still water, about 500 ml, over a 1-1.5 hour session.

3. Try **not to worry** if you miss one day completely but remember if you feel tired after work then a session in the gym will greatly re-vitalise you (really).

4. **Muscles adapt** to the same exercise done for week after week so hit the same muscle group with an **alternative exercise** every few weeks.

5. It is very tempting to use heavier and heavier weights after too short a time-the **"MATCHO (macho) EFFECT"** (i.e. desire to **"match" others lifting big weights in the gym)**. Make sure your **form (your technique) is correct** before you move up the weight otherwise injury can occur.

6. **Do not exercise** if you have a **cold or are ill** as your body is using all its resources to fight the infection and an additional drain on energy sources could be dangerous or even fatal.

7. **Do not exercise shortly after a meal** (within about 1 hour) as all your blood is being used to digest the food rather than being available to the muscles for a sudden workout.

8. **If you feel unwell then stop.** If you still feel unwell some time later consult a doctor.

9. **Do remember to adjust your diet** when you begin training or else you could just stimulate your appetite and put on weight. Again, seek advice from the instructor.

CHAPTER 3

EXERCISE

Alternative Types of Exercise For Gym Haters

These can be undertaken by both **gym-lovers and gym-haters** and have the advantage of reducing or eliminating the need to do aerobic workouts in the gym. The choice of exercises available is enormous and these are summarized in the Table 1 (below) together with the rate at which they burn calories. **Always remember that these figures will vary according to your weight and to the intensity with which you execute the exercise.**

Table 1. ROUGH GUIDE TO CALORIES USED IN VARIOUS TYPES OF EXERCISE BY DIFFERENT WEIGHT PEOPLE.[a]

TYPE OF EXERCISE	CALORIES USED PER HOUR WEIGHT (kilos)		
	60	**86**	**102**
Gym Activities			
AEROBICS-low impact	359	510	605

BOXING-sparring	575	821	968
CIRCUIT TRAINING	511	730	860
CROSS TRAINING MACHINE	492	700	829
CYCLE MACHINE	447	638	753
ROWING-MACHINE	447	638	753
TREADMILL	492	700	829
SKIPPING-fast	638	912	1075

Exercise

WEIGHTS-general	184	261	309
WEIGHTS-vigorous	383	547	645
Sports and Hobbies			
BADMINTON [a]	567	805	954
BASKETBALL [a]	511	730	860
CYCLING	511	730	860
DANCING-ballroom	271	386	457
DANCING-modern aerobic	362	514	609

GOLF-carrying bag	325	474	560
HORSERIDING	255	365	430
MARTIAL ARTS	603	857	1017
ROLLERBLADING	447	638	753
ROWING	638	907	1075
RUGBY [a]	606	862	1021
RUNNING-jogging	599	850	1008
SKIING-cross country	487	692	820

Exercise

SKIING-downhill	391	556	659
SOCCER [a]	575	821	968
SQUASH [a]	816	1092	1248
SWIMMING [a]	383	547	645
TABLE TENNIS [a]	234	340	403
TENNIS-singles [a]	354	504	597
VOLLEYBALL-beach [a]	511	726	860
VOLLEYBALL-gym	241	343	406
WALKING-briskly	263	374	444
WALKING-strolling	184	261	309
YOGA	239	340	403
Home activities			
CLEANING [a]	383	544	645
CLIMBING STAIRS	543	771	914

COOKING- **preparation**	151	217	257
GARDENING-general b	287	431	484
GROCERY SHOPPING	215	306	363
IRONING	136	193	228
PAINTING	303	431	511
SEX [c]	133	189	224
SLEEPING	55	78	92
WATCHING TV	64	91	108
TYPING IN **COMPUTER**	91	120	203

a. This chart is a general guide since the number of calories you burn will vary according to the intensity of any particular exercise including cleaning. With ball games, this will also depend on your level of expertise and length of rallies or time in play. In addition, the numbers given are those burned by a moderately fit person. Also remember that some of the activities shown, such as sex and climbing stairs, do not usually last for one hour!

b. More active digging and hoeing burn many more calories.

c. Numbers for sex are based on a very optimistic 30 minute session with males burning more calories than females.

THE SNACK WAR

Table 2 explains itself. Many such snacks are not only high in calories but also in harmful fats and gradually reducing these between your main meals would have a significantly beneficial effect on your health by reducing weight and blood pressure. This snack reduction together with an increase or introduction of one or more of the sports in Table 1 **could help avoid many of the diseases associated with aging** such as diabetes and heart attacks. Let us face it, we all eat the odd snack or two and this is no problem if we have a regular exercise routine and our weight is under control.

Table 2. SHOWING THE AMOUNT OF EXERCISE TIME (MINUTES) REQUIRED TO USE UP THE CALORIES PRESENT IN VARIOUS TYPES OF SNACKS [a]

TYPE OF SNACK	CALORIES (fat grams)	WALKING	SWIMMING	CYCLING	RUNNING
Cornish Pasty Ginsters (227g)	599 (40.6)	96	66	49	42

Exercise

TYPE OF SNACK	CALORIES (fat grams)	WALKING	SWIMMING	CYCLING	RUNNING
Danish pastry	287 (17.4)	46	31	24	20
Doughnut, jam, (75g)	252 (10.9)	40	27	21	18
Flapjack choc chip (85g)	350 (15.5)	56	38	29	25
Galaxy king size	432 (25.2)	69	47	36	30
Geobar (35g)	127 (1.8)	20	14	10	9
Go Ahead Yoghurt break/slice	68 (2.0)	11	7	6	5
Kit Kat (42g)	212 (11.0)	34	23	17	15

TYPE OF SNACK	CALORIES (fat grams)	WALKING	SWIMMING	CYCLING	RUNNING
Mars Big One (88g)	449 (17.4)	72	49	37	32
Milk Chocolate Dairy whole nut Cadbury (100g)	545 (35.2)	87	60	45	38
Milk Chocolate Digestive Biscuits-2	168 (8.0)	27	18	14	12
Mince-pie (deep-filled)	247	40	27	20	17
Muesli bar (75g)	131 (11.7)	21	14	11	9
Muffin Blueberry Starbucks (100g)	380 (19)	61	41	32	27

Exercise

TYPE OF SNACK	CALORIES (fat grams)	WALKING	SWIMMING	CYCLING	RUNNING
Muffin Chocolate Galaxy (86g)	390 (21.8)	62	42	33	28
Pizza Slice Hawaiian	290 (11.0)	47	32	24	20
Popcorn toffee (100g)	408 (7.2)	65	44	34	29
Pot Noodles beef and tomato	378 (14.0)	61	41	31	27
Potato crisps Walkers 50g	263 (14.5)	42	29	22	19
Potato fries (100g)	294 (14.8)	47	32	24	21
Salted Peanuts(50g)	311 (26.5)	50	34	26	22

TYPE OF SNACK	CALORIES (fat grams)	WALKING	SWIMMING	CYCLING	RUNNING
Sandwich egg and bacon 2 pack	541 (31.3)	87	59	44	38
Sandwich tuna cucumber 2 pack	324 (10.2)	52	36	27	23
SnickersBig One (100g)	501 (28.1)	80	55	41	35
Special K bar (24g)	90 (1.7)	14	10	7	6

a. Based on a someone weighing 86 kilos

Some of the snacks in Table 2 could be substituted, for example by:

1. Fresh or dried fruit (eg. bananas, raisins, sultanas, apricots, prunes, but go easy on the apricots as too many may upset the stomach, also watch out for sulphite preservatives in dried fruit which aggravate allergies). Dates are excellent as they are salt and fat-free but high in fibre, B-vitamins and natural sugar for energy. Each date only contains about 23 calories.

2. A handful of nuts or sunflower or pumpkin seeds (but no more).

3. Unsweetened fruit juice (one glass).

4. Skimmed milk.

5. Small bowl of plain, high fibre, low sugar cereal such as Shredded Wheat, Weetabix or oatmeal with skimmed milk and/or fruit.

6. Plain low fat yoghurt (organic from Sainsbury's is fantastic) with some blueberries, strawberries etc is delicious. Beware of some flavored fruit yoghurts that may contain the artificial sweetener, aspartame, which has recently been reported to induce cancer (see, Table 3 in Chapter 5 of IYL, for details). Frozen yoghurt is a substitute for ice-cream.

7. Boiled eggs occasionally.

8. Rye bread or Ryvita with reduced fat/sugar spread or Marmite.

9. Whole grain, low fat crackers with reduced fat cheese or cottage cheese.

10. Popcorn (98% fat free) or nachos or half a bagel with low fat dip/cheese.

11. Fingers of raw vegetables dipped in low fat dips like hummus etc.

Cravings for sweet snacks may be due to low blood sugar (glucose) resulting from a missed breakfast. Always eat breakfast and include food, such as porridge, cereal or wholemeal toast that release glucose slowly into the blood.

NOW LET'S BEGIN TO EXERCISE

TRUE STORIES SHOWING HOW **NOT** TO BEGIN

Case 1

Is a middle-aged man of 42 who had never been interested in the gym or sport but had begun to put on weight around his waist. He decided to start running to control his weight gain. He failed to ask advice regarding a training schedule but just put on his daps and took off at **high speed** down the hill outside his home. After about one mile, he turned around and started running uphill back to his house. He eventually arrived home exhausted and gasping for breath. The next day massive stiffness set in and he could hardly walk. This was such a traumatic experience that he **never ran** or tried any active exercise again up to now, 15 years later.

Case 2

Involved a 34 year old man who decided to play squash after a **two year lay-off**. The game was very competitive and shortly after finishing he complained of pins and needles in his arms and was unable to breathe properly. He ended up in hospital only to be told by the doctor that another man had died a few days previously on the same squash court! Fortunately, he recovered but **never again participated** in any active sport.

The moral of these stories is to **BEGIN SLOWLY** and select activities that you enjoy and that will retain your enthusiasm. The idea is to increase your daily physical activity not to break a world record. What exactly was the purpose of the runner in Case 1 above? He failed to achieve anything although he could possibly have set a new world speed record for having a heart attack!

THE SENSIBLE WAY

Select some activity that you have or previously had **an interest** in. This could include:

1. Joining a football, rugby, running, tennis, bowls or cycling club – anything to keep you away from the television couch.

2.   Qualifying as a football or rugby referee or coach.

3.   Learning or improving your swimming or gaining a diving qualification which will open a whole new world to you under the sea.

4.   **OR just increasing an activity that you are already involved in** such as walking the dog more often or for a longer time at a faster pace. A study showed that a 20 minute walk with the dog 5 times per week can result in weight loss of 14 lbs in one year. Walking is easy as you need no special training or equipment, although a good pair of shoes/trainers is essential, and you are unlikely to suffer injury. Since many people are goal orientated then why not buy a pedometer to motivate you to achieve the recommended 10,000 paces per day?

Whatever activity you chose, try and involve a friend as, like the "gym buddy" (in Chapter 2), you can motivate each other on a cold dark night to leave the house and exercise. After all, friends are excellent for motivating us to go and drink in the pub.

Some people who hate both exercise and the gym have found that buying a pull-up bar over the door, some dumb-bells and an aerobic workout machine, such as a treadmill or a cycle/rowing machine, for their homes is the answer. If you are a novice to using this equipment then ask a friend for help or enroll for a free induction week at a nearby gym. A good animated website for dumbbell workouts at home is **www.sport-fitness-advisor.com/dumbbellexercises.htm/**. The advantages and disadvantages of the aerobic machines are:

- Their use is independent of the weather

- You can watch the television

- You can record the time, distance, calories burned and pulse rate each day and monitor your progress

- **However,** I have noticed that after a while, these machines tend to become "invisible" and disappear into the rest of the furniture or end up rusting on the patio!

- There are also many other distractions at home such as children, pets, housework etc.

It is up to you to decide whether you wish to confine your exercise to the home or bite the bullet and expose your body to the outside world

Probably, an important consideration is **your location**. Thus, if you live in a dangerous inner city and cannot stand the gym then you have little choice but to remain at home unless you are prepared to drive out of town. On the other hand if, like me, you are lucky enough to live by the sea then you can feel safe in the company of other joggers running along the promenade.

The other advantage of exercising outside is that you will soon see other people jogging with **worse** weight/fitness problems than yourself.

How many times per week?

As mentioned above (see Chapter 2 on the GYM), exercising three times per week for at least 30 minutes is a realistic goal just for the aerobic part of your programme. **DO REMEMBER,** however, that although cycling, running, and football will tone your legs, stomach, heart and lungs, they will do little to maintain your **upper body musculature** and retain a balanced physique. That is why many athletes and sports people include some sort of weight training that not only balances their physiques but also strengthens the whole body and improves their overall performance.

I have often seen it recommended to exercise five times per week (by Medical Officers, no less) to ward off ill-health and obesity. Yes, exercising every day would be ideal but we have to be realistic and set achievable goals. Starting any new programme of exercise, even once or twice per week, is a major effort for some people so let us aim for three sessions per week and take it from there. Three exercise sessions combined with some of the dietary recommendations made above (see Chapter 1 of IYL) will rapidly produce results and be self-fulfilling. It will not only produce pleasing and obvious physical changes but also increased mental alertness and feelings of well-being. These in turn will reinforce the benefits of a new life style and help avoid slipping back to previous self-destructive ways. In addition, trying to exercise five or more times per week will often involve major changes to daily routines, in already busy lives, that are impossible to maintain.

Also, the **amount of exercise required** will depend upon your age, weight, calorie intake and your present level of activity each day. **It is possible to increase** your exercise level each day simply by using the stairs instead of the lift, by walking/cycling into work or by cleaning the house more regularly.

Do remember that exercise will stimulate your appetite

Case 3

I have a number of friends with weight problems who regularly exercise but never seem to shed their "pot bellies". Only by following their eating and drinking habits did I find out why. One friend was very fond of Indian meals and after exercising went to the local Indian restaurant which served "all you can eat" dinners. I joined him on several occasions and although I burnt twice as many calories as him in the gym, he ate **twice as much food as I did!** Another friend regularly ran 3-4 times per week for at least 30 minutes per day. He always seemed to be on the treadmill covered in sweat. He weight trained too but always looked out-of-condition in the changing room. His problem was simply that the exercise seemed to be stimulating his thirst for beer which he drank in large amounts many an evening. One pint of lager with about 200 calories would have taken him at least 15 minutes to jog away and I am sure that he had more than just 2-3 pints in a night.

CHOICE OF DIFFERENT EXERCISES AND SPORTS

The choice of different exercises available seems almost endless but some of the most common ones are listed in Table 1 (above) and the basic characteristics of the most common exercises are given in Table 3 (below). These exercises seem to fall into various categories, namely:

1. Team sports such as rugby, soccer, volleyball, hockey, cricket and basketball

2. Individual or doubles sports such as badminton, squash, tennis, table tennis, cycling, walking, running, skiing, horse riding, swimming, surfing, rollerblading, martial arts, yoga and golf

3. Hobbies/housework such as gardening, cooking, cleaning, decorating and shopping

4. Sex

5. Exercise for lazy or hectic people

1. Team Sports (Table 3)

Most of these are ideal for maintaining fitness of people in their teens, 20s and 30s and up to the beginning of middle age. **I leave individuals to decide when middle age begins!** In contact team sports, especially such as rugby, soccer and basketball, the time to look around for alternative ways to stay fit is usually indicated by recurrent injuries that take ages to heal. Older rugby players sometimes recognize the march of time and play a modified game called "touch rugby" with none of the usual vigorous body tackling allowed.

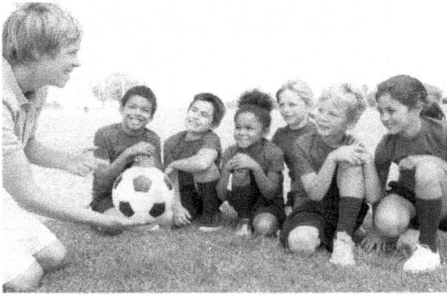

Rugby, soccer and basketball

These require high levels of all-round fitness involving sprinting and high levels of endurance. Different degrees of fitness are required according to the position played. Rugby, soccer and basketball players all benefit from strength training involving weights. With rugby, the emphasis is on all round power, strength and flexibility involving bench pressing and squats. Soccer and basketball players also train with weights to strengthen their legs and maximize vertical jumping ability. Care must be taken not to lose leg strength during endurance training.

Exercise

2. Common Individual or Doubles Sports (Table 3)

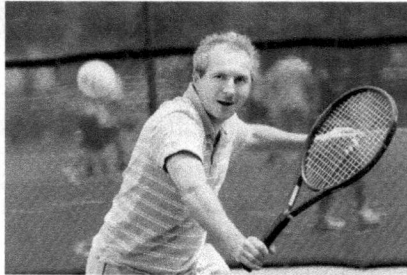

Racket sports

Badminton, squash, tennis and table tennis are sports that can be taken up as children and continued throughout life, even into the 70s and beyond. Care must be taken to avoid injuries to the joints caused by incorrect footwear or racket grip as well as injuries to the eyes or head from squash balls or rackets. Warm-up and warm-down routines are also essential to avoid muscle and joint problems. **Squash, in particular, can be extremely strenuous** and should not be played by unfit, overweight, middle–aged people, new to the sport, without clearance from the doctor.

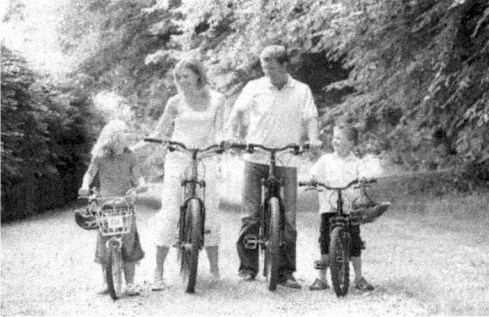

Cycling

This is the most wonderful and exhilarating sport/past-time undertaken by young and old alike. It has the advantage over walking and running in that greater distances are covered more rapidly and the frequent scenery changes maintain interest. Cycling is also a practical replacement for the car/local transport for travelling to work. An even more important advantage of cycling is that it is a low-impact activity that **does little damage to the joints**. Cycling is weight bearing when standing on the pedals for riding up hills (refer to Table 3). Disadvantages are the increased risk of accidents and pollution on busy roads. In addition, there are reports that too frequent cycling for long distances can cause fertility and impotence problems. Reduced sperm counts may result from overheating of the testicles in tight shorts and temporary impotence may be caused by constant pressure from the saddle decreasing the blood flow to the penis. Reduction in excessive bike riding has been advised, in some cases, during attempts to start a family. Padded, gel-containing seat covers offer protection too. Make sure that you cycle about 5 times the distance that you would walk or run. Ensure that you maintain a rhythm sufficient to raise your pulse but can still answer questions from companions-the so-called **"talk-test"**. Finally, do not cycle for a few days prior to the "prostate specific antigen" (PSA) test, which should be undergone by all 50+ year old males every year, as cycling can elevate PSA levels.

Walking

We all walk every day but simply by increasing your walking time each day you can increase your fitness level. Walking is also low impact and weight bearing to strengthen the bones (Table 3). Walk to the shops or to work and take the children to school on foot rather than by car. Walking the dog or with a friend are great ways of increasing your daily exercise. Many of my friends walk to work or at lunchtime and have noticed the difference in their fitness levels after just a few weeks, even though they do no other form of exercise. Recently, it has been recommended that we aim for 10,000 steps each day. Frankly, this sounds ridiculous for busy people to achieve but apparently most people already take 3-5,500 steps per day. I believe that the weather in the UK does not encourage walking but buying a pedometer to record the daily steps can motivate some people. **The 10,000 steps correspond to the minimum level required per day to achieve the benefits of regular exercise.** Some people will prefer to walk indoors on a treadmill away from the rain and cold and can easily record their progress while watching the TV. Gradually increase the time and pace at which you walk and remember the **"talk-test"** to monitor your work intensity. Make sure that you have comfortable shoes appropriate for the terrain.

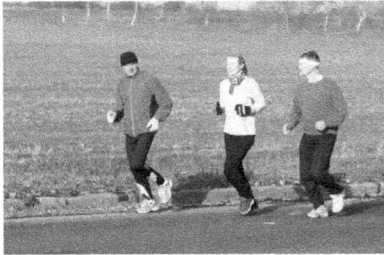

Running and jogging

Running is probably **the most effective way of achieving cardiovascular fitness** and is a major component of many sports. In addition, running at a slower speed (jogging) can be utilized by itself to achieve maximal fitness. Like walking, you can easily adjust your programme to suit your needs and can jog when and where you please. Some people begin by jogging short distances after years of inactivity and end up running marathons! The great advantage of jogging is that it burns calories more rapidly than walking and takes less time. The disadvantage of jogging is that it is **high impact (Table 3) and without good running shoes can damage the joints, especially if you are overweight**. When starting, after years of inactivity, consult your doctor before you begin. If you are unfit and overweight then begin by walking for a short time and then gradually increase your speed until you can run slowly and maintain a conversation **(talk test again)**. Do not worry if progress is slow, but aim to build up the time rather than the distance run, until you can run 20-30 minutes for three times per week. **Do remember to jog in a safe area frequented by other people and try and vary your routine.** Ideally, use a sports centre and run with other people at about the same level of fitness as yourself. Always warm up slowly before running and stretch afterwards.

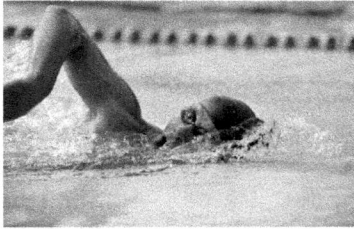

Swimming

Is a marvellous form of general exercise and works out almost **every major muscle group** in the body and increases stamina, strength and flexibility. Swimming also has **low impact** as the water supports the body and there is little stress on any of the joints. Since swimming is not a weight-bearing exercise (Table 3), it does little to strengthen the bones and protect against osteoporosis. It is therefore a good idea to **combine swimming with some weight-bearing exercise** such as walking, running or gym work (Table 3). Swimming is also a good fat-burning exercise and is ideal for people with arthritis, back problems and degenerative diseases as well as pregnant women. The water supports the body, reduces the body weight and allows people to exercise who would normally not be able to because of problems with their joints and back. Swimming is also **excellent for the heart and lungs** since increasing your speed will result in a superb aerobic workout that can easily be undertaken 3 or more times per week. Varying the stroke from backstroke to crawl to breaststroke will also ensure that the majority of muscles in the body are exercised. The value of exercising in water is reflected by the use of swimming pools by many hospital physiotherapists for the treatment of patients with arthritic and other conditions. Regarding the use of swimming for weight loss, there is evidence that swimming is less effective than running or cycling for reducing weight. This may be related to swimming enhancing appetite more than most aerobic activities due to the cooling affect of the water on the body. Again, it is obvious that **all exercise will stimulate the appetite and this urge to eat more has to be controlled.**

Final Comment on Sports

The above sports have the greatest appeal for people wishing to get fit at all ages. This is due to the lack of specialist training required, in most cases, to participate and the wide availability of places to undertake them. **Not all of these activities are suitable for everyone** as evidenced, for example, by my own inability to master swimming beyond a couple of lengths of frantic activity to stay afloat! The important thing is to **find an activity that you enjoy and which you are happy to do three or more times per week** in order to remain fit. Many other sports, such as rowing and skiing, have not been detailed as they require specialist training, equipment or facilities.

3/4. Hobbies/Housework and Sex (Table 3)

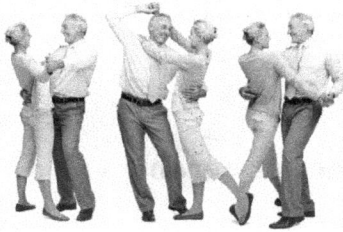

Dancing

Probably one of the **best hobbies** for obtaining and maintaining fitness for the very young and into old age is dancing. Dancing includes ballroom, ballet, square, disco, jazz, jiving, pole and Latin American as well as belly dancing and aerobic workouts, all of which **greatly benefit the heart and lungs and improve flexibility, co-ordination, strength and stamina (Table 3)**. Dancing is also very sociable and helps to find friends and partners. Many events for single people often involve regular meetings for dancing and talking. It was a great relief for me and many of my friends when **disco dancing finally arrived**, as it allowed us to participate without the need to learn prescribed steps or have any degree of co-ordination. Thus, without any training, you can meet members of the opposite sex, have aerobic conditioning and tone the body. The disadvantages include the fact that **many people drink and smoke (not in UK now)** at dance venues. In discos, women also usually benefit more than men who tend to huddle together in groups watching the women!

Exercise/dance or aerobic videos

These videos are also helpful for people (usually women) who **hate the gym or exercising outdoors and prefer to exercise at home**. You can find videos for any type of work-out from yoga to aerobics and dance. Beware videos made by show-biz, usually female, celebrities who have dropped a few dress sizes and are trying to make a fast buck. One of the most ridiculous videos was made by a soap star who lost weight and made a video, then put the weight back on, only to shed it again and make another video! Remember, many videos available are made by fit, good-looking, young women who, lets face it, should be fit at their age. Look under **www.videofitness.com** for a review of videos but **beware those using rapid, high impact, step aerobics**, as without careful instruction on speed, technique and step height, you can easily injure knees and other joints.

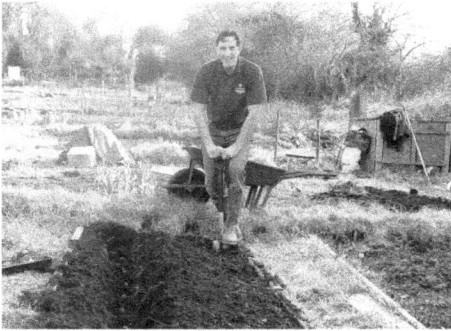

Gardening

Gardening can be a wonderful way of keeping fit but only if activities are included to elevate the pulse and breathing rates (Table 3). It is no use just sowing a few seeds or pruning the roses and expecting to stay fit. In order to stimulate the heart rate, try mowing the lawn using a manual lawn mower, aerating the lawn manually with a fork or digging the vegetable patch. Sawing and chopping are also excellent exercises that can be incorporated. Apart from the fact that it is outside, the great advantage of gardening is the huge satisfaction and health benefits of harvesting your own vegetables and fruit, as well as the sheer pleasure of viewing that well-trimmed lawn and colourful flower beds.

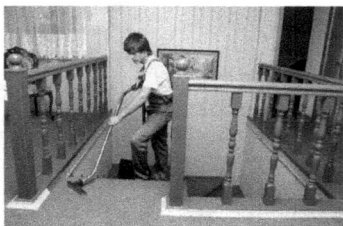

Housework

Personally, I can think of nothing worse than having to rely on housework to assist in remaining fit. It is possible, however, for parents with jobs, and little spare time, to incorporate housework into their fitness programme. Such activities as vacuuming, scrubbing, washing and climbing the stairs will raise the pulse and can be executed with some background music to help maintain a rhythm and pass the time. Remember to elevate the heart rate for at least 20 minutes for optimal effects.

Sex

There is no disputing that exercise is good for the sex life but sex is unlikely to make a major impact on your fitness programme. Regular exercising increases strength, stamina and flexibility all of which will benefit your sex life. In addition, exercise stimulates the release of testosterone and enhances the sex drive. Men who exercise and control their weight also have more active sex lives and less erectile problems.

Table 3. BASIC CHARACTERISTICS OF DIFFERENT EXERCISES

Exercise	Ideal ages	Cardio vascular training	Weight-bearing	Im-pact	Joint dam age	Other injuries	Advan-tages/ Disad-vantages
Teams, rugby, soccer etc	Teens - 30s	Very good	Yes, variable	Yes	Com mon	Very common	Injuries accumu-late
Racket sports	Any	Very good	Yes, legs	Yes	Very com mon	Some-times	Joint wear and tear
Cycling	Any	Very good	Yes, if standing	Low	Low	May reduce fertility	Great distances, pollution/ accident risks
Walking	Any	Fair	Yes, legs	Low	Low	Uncom-mon	Slow but favored by elderly

Exercise

Exercise	Ideal ages	Cardio vascular training	Weight-bearing	Im-pact	Joint dam age	Other injuries	Advan-tages/ Disad-vantages
Run-ning/ jog-ging	Teens to 40 / 50s	Very good	Yes, legs	High	Com mon	Uncom-mon	Safety problem in cities
Swim ming	Any	Very good	No	None	None	Uncom-mon	May also need weight bearing exercise
Danc-ing	Any	Low-Variable	Yes, legs	Yes	Vari-able	Uncom-mon	Sociable but smoking and drinking
Gar-dening	20s +	Low-Variable	Yes, variable	Yes	Vari-able	Cuts	Outside, relaxing, produces vegeta-bles/ flowers
House work	20s +	Low-Variable	Yes, variable	Low	Vari-able	Some-times	Boring, can be danger-ous

OR IS THE FOLLOWING YOU?

5. Exercise for Lazy, Stressed or Hectic People

Despite the vast media exposure of the benefits of a weekly exercise programme, **many people still do very little each day**.

Figure 1. Man overcome by laziness and unaware of long-term harm of his inactive lifestyle

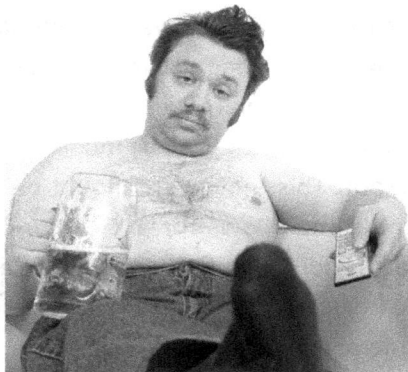

This lack of exercise may be due to:

- **laziness** and lack of concern about their health

- **depression** or excessive stress associated with family/financial problems

- **extremely hectic** lifestyles

The Chartered Association of Physiotherapy have produced an excellent booklet entitled "**The Lazy Exercise Guide**" that may help these groups of people (see reference 137). This booklet explains how daily activities can be modified to provide some sort of workout. **This, however, should be seen only as a stop-gap until time allows for a more organized exercise programme.** In addition, the advice below is also valuable for people who regularly work out. The guide is divided into sections some of which are modified here:

1. **Beginning the day** use the towel to dry your back diagonally from hip to shoulder to provide both a stretch and muscular toning. Stretch legs, arms and neck while dressing.

2. **Journeying** to work in the car and sitting with a straight back and exercising the pelvic floor muscles (abdominal workout and may reduce impotence in men too (see reference 138). On the bus or train, adjust the posture with shoulders back, tummy in and stand as tall as possible. Also, get off one stop earlier and walk to and from work, using the stairs instead of the lift whenever possible in work.

3. **In work** leave your desk every 20 minutes and walk around and stretch the back and legs.

4. **Lunching,** some people use this time for fresh air and a walk, maybe bringing in sandwiches (healthy home made!) and walking to the park. Again concentrate on your posture and walk tall pulling in the tummy.

5. **At home,** walk around or up and down the stairs at every TV commercial break or get up from the computer every 20 minutes. Try and sit upright and support your back at all times. You can also practice pelvic floor exercises while watching TV.

6. **Housework,** activities such as vacuum cleaning, dusting and ironing provide excellent opportunities for additional exercise. Move the furniture around but make sure that you bend your legs when lifting. Play some music and clean in time to this with long sweeping movements and again with the tummy drawn in.

7. **Social events,** again much of the above apply when travelling by car or public transport. It is an excellent idea to try and walk home after a meal rather than catching a taxi. This will help digestion and sleeping.

All the above sounds slightly ridiculous but is just trying to help you to begin some exercise before it is too late. In reality, if you are that lazy or depressed nothing will motivate you and you will not be reading this book.

EXERCISING AT DIFFERENT AGES

It cannot be stated too strongly just how **vitally important it is to undertake some form of exercise throughout life** in order to maintain both physical and mental health. Recent research has shown that as well as the general population, children from **the age of 2 and even people in their 70s, 80s or even 90s benefit** as well as Alzheimer's patients. As mentioned previously, the type of exercise undertaken will vary according to your age.

• Children

Numbers of obese children has risen steadily over the last 20-25 years. A 2005 report from the Governments Information Statistics Division revealed that Scottish children were the fattest in the world with 34% overweight and nearly 20% obese. The later, 2007-2009, rates are very similar for children in the whole UK with 32.6% overweight and 18.3% obese at

10-11 yrs old, and seem to have peaked in the last few years (see reference 139). Unfortunately, overweight and sedentary children tend to develop into overweight adults. These in turn will have higher incidences of bowel cancer, high blood pressure, heart attacks, strokes and type 2 diabetes. The problem of being overweight/obesity needs to be **tackled in children less than 11 years of age before a pattern of poor diet and lack of exercise is developed**. Over 40% of children more than 6 years old may not be exercising for the 30-60 min per day recommended. This is because of the vast amount of time spent in front of the TV and computer, and due to the fact that they do not walk to school or participate regularly in sport.

Increase your children's exercise by:

1. Walking with them to the shops.

2. Buying them a bicycle or skates.

3. Taking them regularly to the park for soccer, basket-ball, cricket etc.

4. Teaching them to swim in the local sports centre.

5. Buying them a dog but only if they agree to walk it every day.

6. Finding out about the amount of physical activity and sport offered at school and becoming involved as a volunteer coach, referee, sponsor etc.

7. Reducing the amount of time they use the computer or spend watching the television each day.

8. Acting as a role model and regularly exercising your-self.

You may soon find that your children's school work, mental health, weight and sleep patterns improve. You too will get more exercise on the touchline or out with the dog.

• Teens and twenties

These are the optimal ages for the type of exercise demanding explosive muscular movements and contact sports. The body is more resilient and flexible and less likely to suffer injury. When injury does occur, the healing process is much more rapid than at later ages. Thus, this is the **best time for soccer, rugby, boxing, skiing, gymnastics, martial arts, basketball and many athletics events**, and is the reason that professionals in most of these sports peak by the time they are 30. This does not mean that the average person should not pursue these sports after 30 but, if they do, then they will be more prone to injury.

Many men in their twenties, who do not participate in the above- mentioned sports, tend to **neglect their cardiovascular workouts** and head for the gym to heave heavy weights around. Reasons for this are fuelled by pressure from society to have the perfect physique both for self fulfillment and for the attraction of the opposite sex. This is apparent from the role models seen in pop videos in which the men with bulging muscles are often surrounded by scantily dressed women. This would be fine if it was not for the great temptation to take shortcuts offered by steroids that are now widely used in some gyms.

This age-group should therefore ensure that they incorporate sufficient aerobic exercise into their gym routines in the form of team sports and/or running, cycling outdoors or aerobic machine work in the gym.

In this age group, particularly, both men and women need to develop an exercise regimen as part of their normal daily routine. Exercise will then be seen as a normal component of their lifestyle and incorporated into later years with minimal effort. This is vitally important since during the late twenties, if not before (see below, "Sarcopenia", for more details), muscles that are not regularly exercised will begin to shrink and fat deposits will begin to build up.

Not as many women as men participate in team sports, and gyms often contain many more men than women. Unfortunately, some women have also adopted men's drinking habits without offsetting these bad habits with regular exercise regimes. The consequences are obvious with increasing numbers of young women overweight.

- ## Thirties to forties

This is the time during which contact sports become replaced with exercises designed to retain physical strength and optimal cardiovascular functioning.

> There are two particular problems that can become apparent after
> 35-40 years of age. These are:

1. Loss of muscle mass – called **"sarcopenia** – (see Figure 2, below) which results in increasing weakness and frailty (see reference 140). It has been estimated that after 45 years old, muscle mass declines about 0.5-1% per year up to 60. Muscle loss then accelerates throughout the 60s, 70s and 80s, and, eventually, results in frailty and the inability to carry out simple daily tasks.

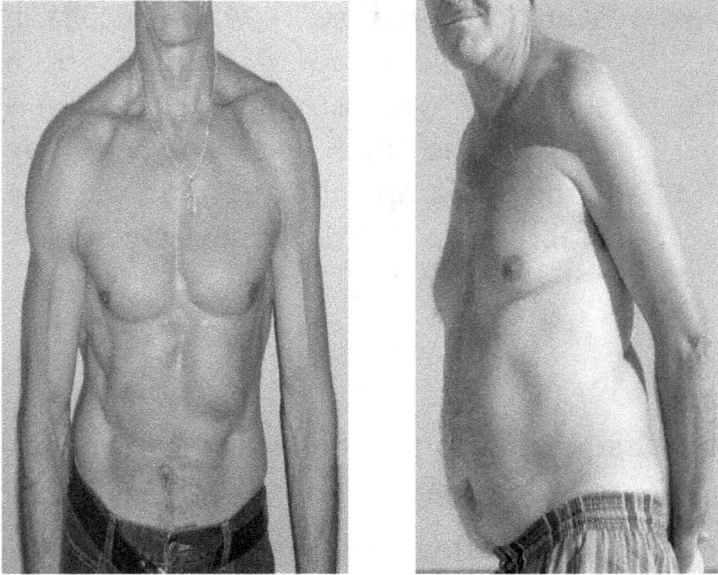

Figure 2. Showing the bodies of two middle aged men. In the right hand photo, it is obvious that some loss of muscle mass has occurred in the upper arms and shoulders and that muscle has been replaced by fat elsewhere. The man in the left photo has used weights to prevent the effects of sarcopenia.

2. Thinning and weakening of the bones — called **"osteoporosis"** — which results in increased likelihood of fractures from minor falls. With osteoporosis, calcium is lost from the bones and if the vertebrae of the spine are affected, and become compressed, then people can shrink remarkably in height.

Both sarcopenia and osteoporosis can, however, be prevented, at least partially, in the 30-40s with weight-bearing exercises. *The best weight-bearing exercises are those using dumbbells, barbells or resistance machines in the gym.* These can easily be substituted for by doing press-ups or other exercises using the body weight or by buying a set of dumbbells for use in the home. The weights should be used 2 or 3 times per week and at each time 9-10 sets of exercises should be done containing 6 to 10 repetitions in each set.

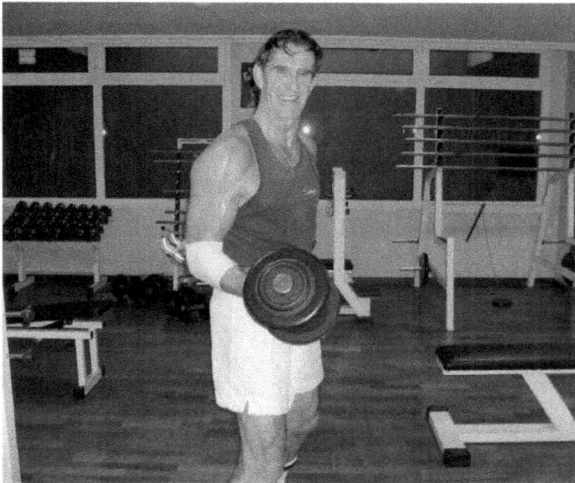

Many men also install a pull-up bar over a doorway which is really excellent for maintaining upper body strength in this age group. Gentler weight-bearing exercises include brisk walking, running, racket sports, skipping, dancing, backpacking, cross-country skiing, volley ball, as well cleaning and digging in the garden. Do these 2-3 times per week for 20-30 min each time. Many of these are excellent as they also provide the required amount of cardiovascular exercise needed each week. The value of swimming as a non-weight bearing, cardiovascular exercise for all ages cannot be over- emphasized but is ineffective at preventing sarcopenia and osteo-porosis.

- **Fifties, sixties and beyond**

Having incorporated exercise into your normal weekly regimen, **there is no reason why this should not be continued into the 50s, 60s and beyond**. There are now more and more people participating in tennis and squash tournaments beyond 65 years old as well as older and older marathon runners reported in the press.

Tennis and walking seem particularly suited for continuation beyond the 60s as they do not require violent bursts of speed and the risk of falls is therefore limited. The normal routines of the younger years can therefore be continued unless overweight, heart disease, high blood pressure, diabetes or arthritis have taken an excessive toll. Hopefully, none of these will apply to readers of this book who have followed the advice offered.

With people living longer, there is more time for them to incorporate regular cardiovascular and weight-bearing exercise into their lives. **Swimming is excellent** for the heart and lungs, and for maintaining flexibility and co-ordination in the older athlete. The value of swimming for the elderly has recently been recognized by Health Challenge Wales and across the UK by the introduction of free swimming for the over 60s. As detailed in the "30s to 40s" section (above), *it is vital to undertake* *resistance training (weight training), as well as exercises for the heart and lungs*, to avoid **sarcopenia or muscle wasting**. Without resistance training, **sarcopenia** will accelerate in the 60s, 70s and 80s resulting in the **"Frailty Syndrome"** with an increasing inability to carry out daily jobs around the house. An elderly person with advanced sarcopenia may even find it impossible to rise from a chair. This physical weakness will lead to disability and dependency on others as routine tasks are neglected. **"The downward spiral of aging" therefore accelerates and the care home will be the only solution as the person can no longer maintain an independent life.**

The important message is that even very unfit elderly people can benefit from an exercise programme, providing there are no major health problems. Unbelievable increases in strength by lifting weights have even been reported for people as old as 90.

IT IS VITAL, FOR MAINTAINING INDEPENDENCE IN OLDER PEOPLE, TO PRESERVE MUSCULAR STRENGTH, CO-ORDINATION AND FLEXIBILITY IN ORDER TO CARRY OUT SIMPLE DAILY TASKS AROUND THE HOME, SUCH AS CLIMBING THE STAIRS, CLEANING AND PREPARING FOOD.

NB. IT IS NEVER TOO LATE TO BEGIN SOME STRENGTHENING EXERCISES – EVEN IN YOUR EIGHTIES

For example, my 86 year old neighbour began exercising, while sitting in her armchair, some very light strengthening exercises for her arms using very small dumbells or weights attached to her wrists with Velcro. After 3 months, she was delighted to be able to lift up her grandchildren to kiss them, for the very first time, as well as to regain her ability to turn her light switches on and off.

Figure 3. Showing the author's elderly neighbour using dumbbells to strengthen arms and shoulders

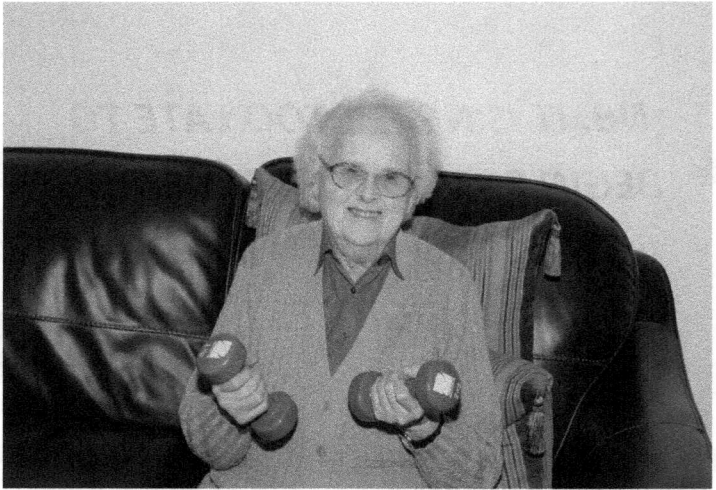

Sarcopenia can, thus, be treated and prevented to a large extent without the use of drugs. These same resistance exercises will also help to protect against osteoporosis (bone thinning).

There is no need to join a gym as light weights are inexpensive to buy and household objects, such as plastic bottles filled with sand or water, are just as effective. A basic home weight resistance programme and exercises for the elderly can be found in reference 141. Such simple programmes not only strengthen the arms, but also the legs in order to prevent falls.

Results can be very impressive with significant increases in both muscle mass and strength recorded even for residents of care homes.

For the complete guide to a healthy life:

It's Your Life: End the confusion from inconsistent health advice

Reference sources for conclusions

Chapter 1

134. Church and Blair, British Journal of Sports Medicine, Vol. 43, pages 80-81, 2009.

135. Kujala, British Journal of Sports Medicine, Vol. 43, pages 550-555, 2009.

136. Hakim and colleagues. Effects of walking on mortality among non-smoking retired men, New England Journal of Medicine, Vol. 338, pages 94-99, 1998.

Chapter 3

137. www.csp.org.uk/uploads/documents/csp_lazy_exercise_lea flet.pdf

138. www.netdoctor.co.uk/pelvicexercise

139. www.ic.nhs.uk/ncmp

140. Schrager, Journal Applied Physiology, Vol. 102, pages 919-925, 2007.

141. www.nia.nih.gov/exercise (click on Chapter 4, "Sample Exercises-Strength")

www.ingramcontent.com/pod-product-compliance
Lightning Source LLC
Chambersburg PA
CBHW050543280326
41933CB00011B/1705